Everything to know about about kidney stones

introduction to Kidney Stones

Introduction:

Kidney stones, also known as renal calculi, are hard deposits that form within the kidneys. These stones can vary in size and shape, ranging from small, sand-like grains to larger, pebble-like structures. Kidney stones are composed of substances such as calcium, oxalate, uric acid, or a combination of these components.

When these substances accumulate in the urine, they can crystallize and clump together, forming kidney stones. The exact cause of kidney stone formation can vary, but factors such as dehydration, diet high in certain minerals, family history, certain medical conditions (such as urinary tract infections or hyperparathyroidism), and certain medications can increase the risk of developing kidney stones.

Kidney stones can cause various symptoms, including severe pain in the back, side, or lower abdomen, pain during urination, blood in the urine, frequent urination, cloudy or foul-smelling urine, and a persistent urge to urinate. However, not all kidney stones produce symptoms and may be incidentally discovered during imaging tests for other reasons.

Although kidney stones can be a common occurrence affecting both men and women, certain preventive measures can help reduce the likelihood of developing stones. Adequate hydration, a balanced diet with moderate intake of salt and animal protein, and avoiding excessive consumption of oxalate-rich foods (such as spinach, beetroot, and chocolate) can be beneficial. Additionally, treating underlying medical conditions that contribute to stone formation and taking prescribed medications as directed can help prevent recurring kidney stones.

If symptoms occur or kidney stones are identified, medical evaluation and treatment may be necessary. Treatment options depend on factors such as stone size, location, and symptoms. Small stones often pass out of the body without intervention and can be managed with pain medication and increased fluid intake. However, larger stones or those causing complications may require medical procedures like lithotripsy (using shock waves to break up the stones), ureteroscopy (using a thin tube to remove or break up the stones), or surgical intervention in some cases.

In conclusion, kidney stones are solid masses formed within the kidneys that can cause discomfort and potentially lead to complications. Understanding the risk factors, preventive measures, and available treatment options is important in managing this condition effectively. If you suspect you may have kidney stones, it is recommended to seek medical advice for proper evaluation and treatment.

TABLE OF CONTENT

Chapter 1…………… Understanding the condition and its causes

Chapter 2…………………………….. symptoms and complications

Chapter 3……………………. Treatment Options and Management

Chapter 4.. Importance of Diet

Chapter 5………………….……. Kidney Stone-Friendly Foods

Chapter 6…………………………… Meal Planning and Recipes

Chapter 7………………………………... prevalence and impact

Chapter 8………………………………… Fluid Intake Strategies

Chapter 9………………………..….. Frequently Asked Questions

Chapter 10……………………………………………Conclusion

Chapter 1

Understanding the condition and it's causes

The development of kidney stones can be attributed to various causes and risk factors, including:

Dehydration: Insufficient fluid intake leads to concentrated urine, which increases the risk of stone formation.

 Diet Consuming a diet high in sodium, oxalate, or calcium can contribute to the formation of certain types of kidney stones. Foods like spinach, chocolate, nuts, and beets contain high levels of oxalate, while excessive salt or calcium intake can lead to calcium stones.

 Family or personal history: Individuals with a family history of kidney stones are more likely to develop them. Additionally, those who have previously had kidney stones are at a higher risk of recurrence.

Certain medical conditions: Medical conditions such as urinary tract infections, cystic kidney diseases, hyperparathyroidism, and certain metabolic disorders like gout or hyperuricemia can increase the risk of kidney stone formation.

Obesity: Being overweight or obese can increase the likelihood of developing kidney stones due to altered hormone levels and dietary factors.

Certain medications: Some medications, such as diuretics, calcium-based antacids, and certain antibiotics, can contribute to the formation of kidney stones.

Age and gender: Kidney stones are more common in adults aged 30 to 60, and men tend to be more affected than women.

Sedentary lifestyle: Lack of physical activity or prolonged periods of sitting can increase the risk of kidney stone formation.

It's worth noting that the causes and risk factors may vary depending on the type of kidney stone. Identification of the specific type of stone through a medical evaluation can help determine the underlying causes and tailor appropriate preventive measures.

- Medical conditions (hyperparathyroidism, urinary tract infections, gastrointestinal disorders)

Here are some medical conditions that may increase the risk of kidney stones and can be affected by consuming oxalate-rich foods like spinach:

1. Hyperparathyroidism: Hyperparathyroidism is a condition in which the parathyroid glands produce excessive amounts of parathyroid hormone (PTH), leading to high levels of calcium in the blood. High blood calcium levels can increase the risk of calcium oxalate kidney stones. In such cases, a low-oxalate diet is often recommended, and spinach consumption may need to be limited.

2. Urinary tract infections: Frequent urinary tract infections (UTIs) can contribute to the formation of struvite stones. These stones may contain calcium, phosphate, and ammonium, and consuming oxalate-rich foods like spinach could potentially worsen the condition and lead to the development of larger stones.

3. Gastrointestinal disorders: Certain gastrointestinal disorders, such as Crohn's disease or short bowel syndrome, can impair the body's ability to absorb oxalate properly. This may result in increased levels of oxalate in the urine, increasing the risk of calcium oxalate kidney stones. In such cases, dietary oxalate restriction, which includes limiting spinach intake, may be advised.

It is essential to note that each person's medical condition and dietary needs can vary. It is always recommended to consult with a healthcare professional or a registered dietitian for personalized advice regarding the dietary management of kidney stones or any other medical condition. They can provide specific recommendations based on an individual's medical history and nutritional needs.
- Dehydration and lack of physical activity
Dehydration and lack of physical activity can have an impact on the formation of kidney stones.

Dehydration: When the body is dehydrated, the urine becomes more concentrated and there is a reduced volume of urine produced. This concentration of urine can lead to the crystallization of substances, such as calcium and oxalate, increasing the risk of kidney stone formation. Therefore, maintaining adequate hydration by drinking enough water throughout the day is essential in preventing kidney stones. Aim for at least 8-10 glasses of water per day, or more if you live in a hot climate or engage in physical activity that causes you to sweat excessively.

Physical activity: Regular physical activity is important for overall health and can also help prevent kidney stone formation. Exercise promotes blood flow and increases the flow of urine, which helps to flush out the kidneys and prevent the accumulation of substances that can lead to stone formation. Physical activity also helps to maintain a healthy body weight, which is important as obesity has been linked to an increased risk of kidney stones. Aim for at least 150 minutes of moderate-intensity aerobic activity, such as brisk walking or cycling, per week.

It is important to note that excessive exercise or intense physical activity without proper hydration can actually increase the risk of kidney stones. This is because intense exercise can lead to increased sweating, which can result in dehydration and concentrated urine. Therefore, it is important to strike a balance between staying physically active and staying adequately hydrated to reduce the risk of kidney stones.

Overall, staying hydrated by drinking enough water throughout the day and maintaining regular physical activity can help prevent the formation of kidney stones. It is always a good idea to consult with a healthcare professional for personalized advice on fluid intake and exercise recommendations based on your individual needs and medical history.

- Diagnosing kidney stones

Diagnosing kidney stones typically involves a combination of medical history, physical examination, and diagnostic tests. Here are some common steps involved in diagnosing kidney stones:

1. Medical History: Your healthcare provider will ask about your symptoms, including the nature, severity, and duration of pain, as well as any urinary or other related symptoms you may be experiencing. They will also inquire about any previous episodes of kidney stones, family history, and any other relevant medical conditions or medications.

2. Physical Examination: A physical examination may be performed to check for any signs of pain or tenderness in the abdomen, back, or sides. The healthcare provider may also examine your lower abdomen and genital areas if your symptoms suggest a possible urinary tract infection.

3. Imaging Tests: The most common imaging tests used to diagnose kidney stones include:

   - X-ray: X-rays can help identify larger kidney stones. However, some types of stones, such as uric acid stones, may not be easily visible on X-rays.

   - Computed Tomography (CT) Scan: CT scans are highly accurate in diagnosing kidney stones. This imaging technique can detect even small stones and provide detailed information about their location, size, and number. It can also help determine if the stone has caused a blockage or any complications.

- Ultrasound: Ultrasound imaging uses sound waves to create images of the kidneys and urinary tract. It can give a preliminary assessment of the presence of kidney stones and their approximate size, but it may not detect very small stones or provide as much detail as a CT scan.

4. Urine Tests: A urine sample may be collected to assess for the presence of blood, infection, and the levels of certain substances that can contribute to stone formation, such as calcium, oxalate, uric acid, and cystine.

5. Blood Tests: Blood tests may be done to evaluate certain parameters like kidney function, calcium levels, uric acid levels, and other blood markers related to stone formation.

6. Stone Analysis: If you pass a kidney stone or it is removed during a medical procedure, your healthcare provider may send it to a laboratory for analysis. The stone analysis can help determine the type of stone, which can guide treatment and prevention strategies.

7. Intravenous Pyelogram (IVP): In this procedure, a dye is injected into a vein, and X-rays are taken as the dye travels through the kidneys, ureters, and bladder. It can provide a detailed view of the urinary tract and identify any abnormalities or blockages caused by kidney stones.

8. Retrograde Pyelogram: This procedure is performed by injecting a dye directly into the ureter through a catheter. X-ray images are taken as the dye travels backward through the ureter, helping to identify any obstructions or abnormalities, such as kidney stones.

9. Magnetic Resonance Imaging (MRI): In certain cases, an MRI scan may be used to evaluate the kidneys and urinary tract. MRI can provide detailed images and can be useful if other imaging techniques are not suitable or if there is a concern about radiation exposure.

Once a diagnosis is made, appropriate treatment options can be discussed. Treatment may vary depending on the size, location, and composition of the kidney stone, as well as the severity of symptoms. It is important to consult with a healthcare professional for an accurate diagnosis and personalized treatment plan.

<u>*Chapter 2*</u>

SYMPTOMS AND COMPLICATIONS

The symptoms of kidney stones can vary depending on the size and location of the stone. Some common symptoms include:

Severe pain: The most prominent symptom of kidney stones is intense, cramping pain in the back or abdomen. The pain may fluctuate in intensity and may radiate to the groin or lower abdomen.

Hematuria: Blood in the urine, known as hematuria, is another typical symptom. It can present as pink, red, or brown urine.

Frequent urination: Needing to urinate more frequently than usual or experiencing an urgent need to urinate is a common symptom.

Cloudy or foul-smelling urine: The presence of kidney stones can cause changes in urine color and odor.

Nausea and vomiting: Some individuals may experience nausea or vomiting as a result of the pain and discomfort caused by kidney stones.

Complications that can arise from kidney stones include:

Urinary tract infections (UTIs): When stones obstruct the urinary tract, it can lead to the development of UTIs, which can cause additional symptoms like fever, chills, and cloudy or foul-smelling urine.

Blockage and kidney damage: Large stones or multiple stones can obstruct the urinary tract and cause a blockage. This blockage can lead to urine backing up into the kidneys, causing kidney damage and potentially leading to kidney failure if not promptly treated.

Hydronephrosis: This condition occurs when the kidney becomes swollen due to a buildup of urine caused by a blockage. Hydronephrosis can cause pain, complications, and damage to the kidney if not relieved.

Recurrent kidney stones: Once an individual has had kidney stones, the likelihood of their recurrence increases. This makes preventive measures crucial in reducing the risk of future stone formation.

If any symptoms of kidney stones are experienced or suspected, it is essential to seek medical attention for proper diagnosis and appropriate treatment.
- Common symptoms of kidney stones (pain, hematuria, urinary urgency)
Common symptoms of kidney stones typically include:

1. Pain: One of the hallmark symptoms of kidney stones is intense pain, often described as severe, sharp, or cramping. The pain is usually felt in the back, side, or lower abdomen. It can come in waves and may fluctuate in intensity as the stone moves within the urinary tract.

2. Hematuria: Kidney stones can cause blood in the urine, a condition known as hematuria. This can result in discolored urine, ranging from pink or red to brown. The presence of blood in the urine may not always be visible to the naked eye and might require a urine test to detect.

3. Urinary urgency and frequency: Kidney stones can irritate the urinary tract, leading to a frequent and urgent need to urinate. Patients may experience a persistent urge to urinate, even if only small amounts of urine are passed.

4. Painful urination: Some individuals with kidney stones may also experience pain or a burning sensation during urination. This discomfort can be attributed to the stone's movement through the ureters, the tubes that connect the kidneys to the bladder.

5. Nausea and vomiting: In certain cases, kidney stone pain can be severe enough to cause nausea and vomiting. These symptoms can occur due to the intense pain or as a result of nerve stimulation caused by the stones.

It is important to note that the severity and combination of symptoms can vary depending on factors such as the size, location, and number of kidney stones present. If you suspect you have kidney stones or are experiencing any of these symptoms, it is recommended to seek medical attention for proper diagnosis and appropriate management.

- Potential complications (kidney damage, urinary tract infection, blockage of urinary flow)

Kidney stones can potentially lead to various complications, including:

1. Kidney damage: The movement or presence of kidney stones can cause harm to the kidneys. If a stone becomes lodged in the urinary tract, it can obstruct the normal flow of urine, leading to increased pressure within the kidney. This increased pressure can impair kidney function, potentially causing kidney damage or kidney failure if not addressed promptly.

2. Urinary tract infection (UTI): Kidney stones can create an environment favorable for bacterial growth within the urinary tract. If the stone obstructs the flow of urine, it can result in stagnant urine, which increases the risk of UTIs. Symptoms of UTIs may include pain or discomfort during urination, foul-smelling urine, frequent urination, and fever. Prompt treatment with antibiotics is necessary to prevent the infection from spreading to the kidneys.

3. Blockage of urinary flow: Larger kidney stones or stones that get lodged in the urinary tract can act as a physical barrier, obstructing or partially blocking the flow of urine. This blockage can cause further pain and discomfort while also impairing the kidneys' ability to eliminate waste products from the body. In severe cases, it may necessitate immediate medical intervention to relieve the obstruction.

4. Hydronephrosis: Hydronephrosis is the backup or swelling of urine within the kidneys due to obstruction. It can occur when a kidney stone blocks the normal flow of urine, causing urine to accumulate and distend the kidney. If left unaddressed, hydronephrosis can cause kidney damage and impair renal function.

5. Kidney infection (pyelonephritis): Obstructive kidney stones increase the risk of developing a kidney infection. Bacteria can ascend from the lower urinary tract and colonize the kidneys, leading to pyelonephritis. This condition is characterized by symptoms such as high fever, chills, flank pain, and general malaise. It requires immediate medical attention and treatment with antibiotics.

It is important to be aware of these potential complications and seek medical intervention if you suspect you have kidney stones or experience any related symptoms. Timely diagnosis and appropriate management can help prevent or minimize the risks associated with kidney stones.

Chapter 3

TREATMENT OPTIONS AND MANAGEMENT

The treatment and management of kidney stones depend on factors such as the size, location, and composition of the stones, as well as the individual's overall health. Here are some common treatment options and management strategies for kidney stones:

Watchful waiting: Small kidney stones (less than 5mm) that are not causing severe symptoms may be managed with pain medication and increased fluid intake to help the stone pass naturally. Regular monitoring with imaging studies is necessary to ensure the stone is not growing or causing complications

Medications: Certain medications may be prescribed to help manage kidney stones, depending on the type and underlying cause. For example, medications like alpha blockers can relax the muscles in the ureter, facilitating the passage of stones. Other medications may be given to control pain, prevent infection, or reduce stone formation.

Extracorporeal Shock Wave Lithotripsy (ESWL): This non-invasive procedure uses high-energy shock waves to break kidney stones into smaller pieces that can be more easily passed through the urinary tract. ESWL is commonly used for stones less than 2cm in size.

Ureteroscopy: This minimally invasive procedure involves passing a thin tube (ureteroscope) through the urethra and bladder to reach and remove or break the kidney stone in the ureter. It is particularly effective for stones located in the lower part of the urinary tract.

Percutaneous Nephrolithotomy (PCNL): This is an invasive procedure performed under general anesthesia. A small incision is made in the back to access the kidney, and a nephroscope is used to remove or break the stone. PCNL is generally used for larger stones or when other treatments have failed.

Dietary and lifestyle modifications: Making certain changes in diet and lifestyle can help prevent the formation of kidney stones or reduce their recurrence. This may include increasing fluid intake, reducing sodium and animal protein consumption, and limiting oxalate-rich foods (e.g., spinach, chocolate).

 Preventive medication: In individuals with recurrent kidney stones or certain underlying conditions, preventive medications may be prescribed to inhibit the formation of new stones. These medications can help control urine composition and decrease the risk of stone recurrence.

The choice of treatment approach depends on multiple factors and should be determined by a healthcare professional based on individual circumstances. It's important for those who have had kidney stones to work closely with their healthcare team to determine the most appropriate treatment and management plan.

- Non-surgical treatment approaches (fluid intake, pain management).

Non-surgical treatment approaches for kidney stones typically involve managing pain and increasing fluid intake to encourage stone passage. Here are some common treatments:

1. Pain Management: Over-the-counter pain medications may be recommended to manage the pain associated with kidney stones. Nonsteroidal anti-inflammatory drugs (NSAIDs), such as ibuprofen or naproxen, can help alleviate pain and reduce inflammation. Your healthcare provider may prescribe stronger pain medications if necessary.

2. Increased Fluid Intake: Drinking plenty of fluids is crucial for kidney stone management. Adequate hydration helps dilute urine and flush out substances that can form stones. Water is the best choice, and you should aim to drink enough to produce clear or light-colored urine. Your healthcare provider may provide specific recommendations based on your individual needs.

3. Medication: Depending on the type of kidney stone you have, certain medications may be prescribed. For example, if you have calcium stones, medications like thiazide diuretics or phosphate solutions may be given to help prevent stone formation. If you have uric acid stones, medications called allopurinol or potassium citrate may be prescribed to decrease uric acid levels or increase urine pH.

4. Extracorporeal Shock Wave Lithotripsy (ESWL): This non-surgical procedure uses sound waves to break kidney stones into smaller fragments that can be passed naturally through urine. ESWL is commonly used for smaller stones that are located in the kidney or upper ureter.

5. Ureteroscopy: This minimally invasive procedure involves passing a thin tube with a camera (ureteroscope) into the ureter to locate and remove or break up the stone. It is often used for stones located in the lower ureter.

- Surgical intervention and procedures (lithotripsy, ureteroscopy, percutaneous nephrolithotomy)

When kidney stones form and cause symptoms such as pain, infection, or obstruction, surgical intervention may be necessary. The choice of procedure depends on factors like the size, location, and number of stones, as well as the patient's overall health.

1. Lithotripsy: This procedure is commonly referred to as Extracorporeal Shock Wave Lithotripsy (ESWL). It uses shock waves to break large kidney stones into smaller pieces, allowing them to pass more easily through the urinary tract. Lithotripsy is non-invasive and performed externally, so there is no need for surgical incisions.

2. Ureteroscopy: A ureteroscope, a long, flexible tube with a camera and light at the end, is inserted into the urethra and passed through the bladder into the ureter. It allows the urologist to visualize the stone and either remove it or break it into smaller fragments with laser energy. Small stones can be removed completely during the procedure, while larger ones may require additional treatments like lithotripsy.

3. Percutaneous Nephrolithotomy (PCNL): This surgical procedure is performed under general anesthesia. A small incision is made in the back, and a nephroscope is inserted directly into the kidney. The stones are either removed intact or crushed with various instruments, and then the fragments are extracted. PCNL is typically used for larger stones or in cases where other procedures are not feasible.

Other less common surgical interventions for kidney stones may include open surgery (nephrolithotomy or pyelolithotomy), which involves making an incision directly into the kidney or renal pelvis to remove stones. These procedures are typically reserved for complex cases or when other treatment options have failed.

The choice of procedure depends on several factors, and it is best to consult with a urologist who can evaluate the individual case and recommend the most suitable treatment approach.

Chapter 4

IMPORTANCE OF DIET IN KIDNEY STONE PREVENTION

Diet plays a crucial role in the prevention of kidney stones. Making certain dietary modifications can help reduce the risk of stone formation and recurrence. Here are some key ways in which diet can be important in kidney stone prevention:

Adequate fluid intake: Drinking plenty of fluids, especially water. Fluid Intake: Adequate fluid intake is essential in the prevention and management of kidney stones. It helps dilute the urine and flush out substances that can form stones. Water is the best choice for hydration. Individuals with a history of kidney stones should aim to drink at least 8 cups (64 ounces) of water per day or more, depending on their activity level and climate.

Limiting sodium intake: High sodium intake can increase the amount of calcium in the urine, which can lead to the formation of calcium-based kidney stones. It is important to reduce the consumption of processed foods, canned soups, and salty snacks, and to opt for low-sodium alternatives.

Moderating animal protein consumption: A diet high in animal protein, particularly red meat, can increase the risk of kidney stone formation. Animal protein can lead to higher levels of uric acid and calcium in the urine, which can contribute to stone formation. It is advisable to consume moderate amounts of lean protein sources, such as poultry, fish, and plant-based protein sources.

Limiting oxalate-rich foods: Some kidney stones are composed of calcium oxalate. Oxalate is found in certain foods such as spinach, rhubarb, beets, and nuts. Limiting the consumption of oxalate-rich foods can help reduce the risk of stone formation. It is important to note that individuals with a history of calcium oxalate stones may need to reduce but not eliminate these foods from their diet.

Choosing a balanced diet: A diet that is balanced and includes a variety of fruits, vegetables, whole grains, and low-fat dairy products can help reduce the risk of kidney stone formation.

These foods provide essential nutrients and help maintain a healthy weight, which is important for kidney stone prevention.

Moderate calcium intake: Contrary to popular belief, calcium-rich foods do not increase the risk of kidney stones. In fact, consuming an adequate amount of calcium from food sources can help bind to oxalate in the intestine, reducing its absorption and lowering the risk of stone formation. It is generally recommended to obtain calcium from food sources rather than supplements.

It is important to note that dietary modifications for kidney stone prevention should be tailored to the individual's specific type of stone and underlying medical conditions. Consulting with a healthcare professional or a registered dietitian can help provide personalized dietary recommendations for kidney stone prevention.

Increase citrate consumption: Citrate helps prevent the formation of certain types of kidney stones. Good dietary sources of citrate include citrus fruits (such as lemons and oranges), melons, and some vegetables like kale and broccoli.

Calcium Intake: Contrary to common belief, consuming an adequate amount of calcium from food sources is important in the prevention of kidney stones. Calcium binds to oxalate in the digestive tract, preventing its absorption and reducing the risk of calcium-based stone formation. However, calcium supplements should be avoided unless specifically recommended by a healthcare professional.

Oxalate Intake: Some types of kidney stones are composed of calcium oxalate. Foods high in oxalate, such as spinach, rhubarb, beets, nuts, and chocolate, should be limited in individuals with a history of calcium oxalate stones. It is important to note that completely eliminating oxalate-rich foods from the diet is not necessary unless advised by a healthcare professional.

Acidic Foods: In some cases, certain kidney stones can be caused by high levels of uric acid or low urinary citrate. Avoiding or limiting foods that are high in purines, such as organ meats, shellfish, and some types of fish, can help reduce uric acid levels. Additionally, consuming citrus fruits and their juices can increase urinary citrate levels, which can help prevent stone formation.

Weight Management: Maintaining a healthy weight is important in preventing kidney stones. Obesity and excessive weight gain can increase the risk of stone formation. Consuming a balanced diet that includes fruits, vegetables, whole grains, and lean protein sources can promote a healthy weight and reduce the risk of kidney stones.

Limit Soda and Sugar-Sweetened Beverages: Regular consumption of soda and sugar-sweetened beverages has been linked to an increased risk of kidney stones. These drinks are high in sugar and can lead to dehydration. It's best to choose water or unsweetened beverages as your main source of hydration.

Limit Oxalate-Rich Foods: If you have calcium oxalate stones, it may be helpful to limit your intake of foods high in oxalate. Some examples of high-oxalate foods include spinach, Swiss chard, beet greens, rhubarb, peanuts, and wheat bran. However, it's important to note that cooking or steaming these foods can help reduce their oxalate content.

. Increase Dietary Fiber: A diet rich in fiber can help reduce the risk of kidney stones. Fiber helps bind to calcium in the digestive tract, preventing its absorption and decreasing the levels of calcium in the urine. Consuming a variety of fruits, vegetables, whole grains, legumes, and nuts can help increase your fiber intake.

Moderate Consumption of Oxalate-Rich Drinks: In addition to food sources, some beverages can also have high oxalate content. Tea, coffee, and some fruit juices like cranberry and orange juice may contain significant amounts of oxalate. However, completely eliminating these beverages is not necessary unless specifically advised by a healthcare professional.

Monitor Protein Intake: If you have a history of kidney stones, it's important to monitor your protein intake, especially animal protein. High intakes of protein can increase the excretion of calcium and uric acid, leading to the formation of stones. Strive for moderation and balance by including plant-based protein sources like legumes, tofu, and tempeh in your diet.

Be Cautious with Supplements: Be cautious when it comes to dietary supplements. Some supplements, like vitamin C and calcium supplements, can increase the risk of stone formation if taken in excess. It's best to talk to a healthcare professional before starting any new supplements.

High-purine foods: Purines are naturally occurring compounds found in some foods, and when they are broken down, they produce uric acid. Uric acid stones can form as a result. Limit your intake of foods high in purines such as organ meats, sardines, anchovies, scallops, and some types of seafood.

Sugar-sweetened beverages: Consuming excessive amounts of sugary drinks like soda, fruit juices, and sweetened iced tea can increase the risk of kidney stone formation. Opt for water, herbal tea, or unsweetened beverages instead
Stay Active: Regular physical activity can help with kidney stone prevention. Exercise promotes healthy weight management, improves digestion, and reduces the risk of certain health conditions that can contribute to stone formation. Aim for at least 150 minutes of moderate-intensity exercise per week.

Limit Alcohol Consumption: Excessive alcohol consumption can increase the risk of dehydration, which can contribute to kidney stone formation. It's best to limit alcohol intake and drink in moderation.

Remember, the recommendations may vary based on the type of kidney stones you have and any underlying health conditions, so it's important to consult a healthcare professional or a registered dietitian for personalized advice. They can help you create a diet plan that suits your needs and supports kidney stone prevention and management..

While it's not necessary to completely eliminate these foods from your diet, limiting your intake of high-oxalate and high-sodium foods may be beneficial in preventing kidney stone formation. Here is a list of foods that are high in oxalate or sodium:

Foods High In Oxalate:

- Spinach
Spinach is known to be rich in oxalate due to its chemical composition. Oxalate, or oxalic acid, is a naturally occurring organic acid found in many plant-based foods. The amount of oxalate differs among different vegetables, with spinach having relatively high levels compared to others.

Here are some key details about why spinach is rich in oxalate:

1. Chemical structure: Spinach contains high levels of oxalate because its chemical structure promotes the formation of calcium oxalate crystals. These crystals can contribute to the development of kidney stones or other health issues in susceptible individuals.

2. Oxalate formation: Spinach plants produce oxalate as a byproduct of metabolism. It is primarily found in the leaves of the plant, which is why spinach leaves are the part commonly consumed.

3. Environmental factors: Oxalate levels in spinach can be influenced by environmental factors such as soil composition and climate. Certain conditions may lead to an accumulation of oxalate in plants, including spinach.

4. Cooking effect: Cooking or boiling spinach can reduce its oxalate content. Studies have shown that boiling spinach lowers its oxalate levels by leaching it into the cooking water. However, this does not mean there will be a significant reduction in oxalate content, so moderation is still advised.

5. Health considerations: While spinach is a nutrient-rich vegetable, individuals with certain health conditions, such as kidney stones, may be advised to moderately restrict their oxalate intake. This precaution is due to the potential for calcium oxalate crystal formation in the urinary tract, which can contribute to the development of kidney stones.

It is important to note that the oxalate content of spinach should not discourage its consumption unless advised otherwise by a healthcare professional. Spinach offers numerous health benefits, including being rich in vitamins, minerals, and antioxidants.

Spinach, being rich in oxalate, may not be recommended for individuals who have a history of kidney stones or are at risk of developing them. This is because calcium oxalate is the most common type of kidney stone, and consuming foods high in oxalate, like spinach, can contribute to their formation in susceptible individuals

- Swiss chard

Swiss chard, like several other leafy green vegetables, contains varying levels of oxalates. Oxalates are naturally occurring compounds found in many foods and can contribute to the formation of kidney stones in susceptible individuals. While Swiss chard is a nutritious vegetable, it is also considered relatively high in oxalates compared to some other leafy greens.

Oxalates are formed when oxalic acid combines with minerals like calcium or potassium in the body. Swiss chard contains significant amounts of oxalic acid, which can bind with calcium and form calcium oxalate, a major component of kidney stones.

It's important to note that not everyone who consumes high-oxalate foods will develop kidney stones, as stone formation is influenced by several factors, including individual predisposition, overall diet and hydration status. However, individuals prone to kidney stones or with a history of oxalate-related health issues should be cautious about their oxalate intake and may need to limit consumption of high-oxalate foods like Swiss chard.

- Beets

Beets, like Swiss chard, also contain oxalates. While the exact oxalate content may vary depending on the beet variety and size, beets can be classified as a food with moderate to high oxalate levels.

Oxalates are naturally occurring compounds that are found in numerous plant foods. They can combine with minerals like calcium to form calcium oxalate, which is a component of kidney stones in some individuals.

Beets contain oxalic acid, which is one of the main components contributing to their oxalate content. Consuming beets, especially in large amounts or frequently, can increase the intake of oxalates.

As with other high-oxalate foods, it's important to note that not everyone who consumes beets will develop kidney stones. However, individuals with a history of oxalate-related health issues or those prone to kidney stones may need to limit their intake of high-oxalate foods, including beets.

- Rhubarb

Rhubarb is another vegetable that is known to contain high levels of oxalates. The oxalate content of rhubarb can vary depending on the specific variety, growing conditions, and cooking methods.

The high oxalate levels in rhubarb are mainly attributed to the presence of oxalic acid, a naturally occurring compound. When consumed, oxalic acid can bind with minerals like calcium or potassium in the body to form calcium oxalate, which is a major component of kidney stones in some individuals.

The leaves of the rhubarb plant are particularly high in oxalates, but the stalks also contain significant amounts. It's important to note that the stalks are typically the only part of rhubarb used in cooking and baking, as the leaves are considered toxic due to their high oxalate content.

Due to its high oxalate levels, individuals with a history of oxalate-related health issues or those prone to kidney stones may need to limit their consumption of rhubarb.

As always, it's best to consult with a healthcare professional or a registered dietitian if you have concerns about your diet and oxalate intake. They can provide personalized guidance based on your specific needs and health conditions.

- Strawberries

Strawberries are a popular fruit that is enjoyed by many. While strawberries are generally considered a nutritious and delicious addition to a balanced diet, they do contain a moderate amount of oxalates.

The oxalate content in strawberries is not as high as in some other vegetables and fruits, but it is still present. The exact oxalate levels can vary depending on the specific variety, growing conditions, and ripeness of the strawberries.

Oxalates are natural compounds found in a wide range of foods, including fruits, vegetables, grains, and even some beverages. When consumed, oxalates can bind with minerals in the body, such as calcium, to form calcium oxalate, which can contribute to the formation of kidney stones in susceptible individuals.

However, it's important to note that the overall oxalate content in strawberries is relatively low compared to other high-oxalate foods like spinach, beets, or rhubarb. Additionally, strawberries are also rich in other beneficial nutrients like vitamin C, fiber, and antioxidants, which make them a valuable addition to a well-balanced diet.

If you have a history of oxalate-related health issues or are concerned about your oxalate intake, it's always a good idea to consult with a healthcare professional or a registered dietitian. They can provide personalized guidance and help you make informed decisions about your diet.

- **Nuts** (such as almonds, cashews, and peanuts)

Nuts such as almonds, cashews, and peanuts generally have moderate oxalate content compared to other foods. The exact oxalate levels can vary, but they are not considered to be very high oxalate foods.

Oxalates are natural compounds found in a wide range of plant-based foods, including nuts. When consumed, oxalates can bind with minerals in the body, such as calcium, to form calcium oxalate, which can contribute to the formation of kidney stones in susceptible individuals.

However, it's important to note that the overall oxalate content in nuts is still relatively low compared to some high-oxalate foods like spinach, beet greens, or rhubarb. Nuts are also packed with beneficial nutrients like healthy fats, protein, fiber, vitamins, and minerals, which make them a nutritious part of a well-balanced diet.

If you have a history of oxalate-related health issues or are concerned about your oxalate intake, it's always a good idea to consult with a healthcare professional or a registered dietitian. They can provide personalized guidance and help you make informed decisions about your diet.

- **Seeds** (such as sesame seeds and poppy seeds)

Seeds, including sesame seeds and poppy seeds, contain varying levels of oxalate. While they are not among the highest oxalate foods, they do contain a moderate amount of oxalates.

Oxalates are naturally occurring compounds found in many plant-based foods. When consumed, oxalates can bind with minerals, such as calcium, in the body and form calcium oxalate, which can contribute to kidney stone formation in some individuals.

Sesame seeds and poppy seeds have several nutritional benefits, including being rich in healthy fats, protein, fiber, vitamins, and minerals. However, if you have a history of kidney stones or are concerned about your oxalate intake, it's important to be aware of foods that contain higher levels of oxalates.

- **Soy products** (such as tofu and soy milk)

Soy products like tofu and soy milk typically have low to moderate oxalate content. While they do contain some oxalates, their levels are generally not considered high.

Oxalates are naturally occurring compounds found in various plant-based foods. When consumed, oxalates can combine with calcium to form calcium oxalate, which can contribute to the formation of kidney stones in susceptible individuals.

However, it's important to note that the overall oxalate content in soy products is relatively low compared to other high-oxalate foods like spinach or rhubarb. Soy products are also known for their nutritional benefits, as they are excellent sources of plant-based protein, essential amino acids, healthy fats, and various vitamins and minerals.

- **Chocolate**
chocolate, while it is not a significant source of oxalate, some types of chocolate, particularly dark chocolate, may contain moderate levels of oxalates. However, in the context of a varied diet, the oxalate content in chocolate is typically not a major concern unless you have specific dietary restrictions or health conditions. Once again, it's best to consult with a healthcare professional for personalized advice.

- **Tea**:
 Tea, particularly black tea, contains moderate levels of oxalates. However, the exact amount can vary depending on factors such as the type of tea and brewing time.

- **Wheat bran:**
 Wheat bran is relatively high in oxalates. It is important to note that bran from other grains, such as rice or oats, may also contain oxalates but at different levels.

- **Quinoa:**
 Quinoa typically contains moderate levels of oxalates. However, the oxalate content can vary among different varieties and how it is prepared.

- **Potatoes:** Potatoes generally have low oxalate content, making them a suitable choice for individuals with concerns about oxalate intake.

- **Okra:**

Okra is considered a low-oxalate food, making it a good choice for those wanting to limit oxalate consumption.

- Celery:
Celery is also classified as a low-oxalate food. It is generally safe for individuals with concerns about oxalate intake.

- Cucumber:
Cucumber is typically low in oxalates, making it a suitable choice for individuals looking to limit oxalate consumption.

Foods High In Sodium:

These foods are high in sodium because they either naturally contain sodium or have added sodium during processing. Here's how each food item listed is high in sodium:

- Processed meats:
Processed meats like deli meats and sausages can be high in sodium due to the addition of salt and other sodium-containing ingredients during processing.

- Canned soups and broths:
Canned soups and broths often have high sodium content to enhance flavor and preserve the product. Sodium is commonly added as a preservative and seasoning.

- Canned vegetables:
Canned vegetables may have added salt or brine, which significantly increases their sodium content.

- Bacon:
Bacon is typically cured with salt or sodium-containing substances, resulting in its high sodium content.

- Pickles:
Pickles are often preserved in a brine solution containing high amounts of sodium, contributing to their sodium content.

- Olives:
Olives are preserved in brine, which contains high levels of sodium.

- Frozen meals:
Frozen meals, especially those that are pre-packaged or processed, often contain high sodium levels as a preservative and flavor enhancer.

- Fast foods:
  Fast food items are often high in sodium due to the use of processed ingredients, salt, and seasoning mixes.

- Salted snacks:
  Salted snacks like chips and pretzels are typically seasoned with salt, leading to their high sodium content.

- Condiments:
  Condiments like ketchup, soy sauce, and salad dressings often have added salt or sodium-containing ingredients.

- Cheese:
  Some types of cheese, particularly processed cheese and certain varieties like feta or blue cheese, can be high in sodium.

- Smoked or cured meats:
  Similar to bacon, smoked or cured meats, such as ham or sausage, often contain added salt or are processed with sodium-containing compounds.

- Salted nuts:
  Nuts can be salted during processing or as a seasoning, resulting in their high sodium content.

It's important to note that everyone's tolerance for these foods and their ability to contribute to kidney stone formation can vary. If you have a history of kidney stones or are at a higher risk, it's a good idea to work with a healthcare professional or a registered dietitian who can provide personalized recommendations. They can help you create a balanced diet plan that takes into account your individual needs and supports kidney stone prevention.

<u>Chapter 5</u>

Kidney stones friendly food

In addition to avoiding certain foods, there are also kidney stone-friendly foods that can help support kidney health and reduce the risk of stone formation. Here's a detailed guide to foods that are low in oxalate and sodium, and high in beneficial nutrients for kidney health:

Calcium-rich foods: Contrary to popular belief, consuming foods rich in calcium can actually help prevent kidney stones. Calcium binds with oxalate in the digestive tract, reducing its absorption and decreasing the risk of stone formation. Good sources of low-oxalate calcium include dairy products like milk, yogurt, and cheese, as well as leafy green vegetables like kale and broccoli.

- **Citrus fruits:** Citrus fruits, such as oranges, lemons, and grapefruits, are high in citrate, which can help prevent the formation of calcium oxalate stones. Citrate helps inhibit the growth of crystals and also increases urine volume, helping to flush out stone-forming substances. Include fresh citrus fruits or drink their juices regularly, but be mindful of the sugar content if you have diabetes or metabolic syndrome.

- **Water:** Staying hydrated is crucial for kidney health and preventing stone formation. Drinking an adequate amount of water helps dilute urine and flush out waste products. Aim to drink at least 8 cups (64 ounces) of water per day, or more if recommended by your healthcare professional.

- **Fiber-rich foods:** Consuming a diet high in fiber can help regulate digestion and promote regular bowel movements, which is important for kidney health. Include plenty of fruits, vegetables, whole grains, and legumes in your diet to increase your fiber intake.

- **Low-oxalate vegetables:** While some vegetables are high in oxalate, there are plenty of low-oxalate options that can be safely included in a kidney stone-friendly diet. These include asparagus, cauliflower, cabbage, cucumbers, bell peppers, zucchini, and lettuce.

- **Low-sodium foods:** Limiting sodium intake is essential to maintain proper fluid balance and reduce the risk of stone formation. Choose fresh and minimally processed foods, and avoid adding excess salt to your meals. Instead, use herbs, spices, and other salt-free seasonings to add flavor.

- **Plant-based proteins:** Incorporating more plant-based protein sources into your diet can help reduce the risk of stone formation. Legumes (such as beans, lentils, and chickpeas), tofu, tempeh, and quinoa are excellent sources of protein without the high levels of purines found in animal proteins.

- **Olive oil: Olive** oil is a healthy fat that can be beneficial for kidney health. It contains monounsaturated fats, which have been shown to have anti-inflammatory properties and may help protect against kidney damage.

- **Herbal teas:** Certain herbal teas, such as nettle leaf tea and dandelion root tea, have been traditionally used to support kidney health and prevent stone formation. These teas have diuretic properties that can help increase urine production and flush out waste products.

- **Low-oxalate fruits:** While some fruits are high in oxalate and should be limited, there are also low-oxalate options that can be enjoyed in moderation. These include berries (such as strawberries, blueberries, and raspberries), apples, pears, and grapes.

- **Herbs and spices:** Seasoning your meals with herbs and spices can add flavor without the need for excess salt. Some herbs and spices, such as parsley, basil, and turmeric, have been traditionally used to support kidney health.

- **Probiotic-rich foods:** Consuming foods that are rich in probiotics, such as yogurt and fermented foods like sauerkraut and kimchi, can help promote a healthy gut microbiome. A healthy gut is important for overall health, including kidney health.

- **Nuts and seeds:** Nuts and seeds provide healthy fats, protein, and fiber, making them a nutritious addition to a kidney stone-friendly diet. Choose unsalted varieties and enjoy them in moderation.

- **Garlic and onions:** Garlic and onions contain compounds that have been shown to have antioxidant and anti-inflammatory properties, which can be beneficial for kidney health. They can be used to add flavor to a variety of dishes.

- **Fish high in omega-3 fatty acids:** Fatty fish, such as salmon, mackerel, and sardines, are excellent sources of omega-3 fatty acids. These healthy fats have anti-inflammatory properties and may help protect against kidney damage.

- **Green tea:** Green tea is rich in antioxidants and has been associated with a reduced risk of kidney stone formation. It may help inhibit the growth of crystals and promote overall kidney health.

- **Watermelon:** Watermelon is not only hydrating, but it also contains high levels of citrulline, which can help increase urine production and prevent the formation of calcium oxalate stones.

- **Red bell peppers:** Red bell peppers are low in oxalate and high in vitamin C, an antioxidant that can help protect against kidney damage. They can be enjoyed raw, roasted, or sautéed.

.

- **Whole grains:** Whole grains like brown rice, quinoa, and whole wheat bread provide fiber and essential nutrients. They can help regulate blood sugar levels and promote heart health, which is important for kidney health as well.

- **Legumes:** Legumes such as beans, lentils, and chickpeas are high in fiber, protein, and various vitamins and minerals. They can be a good plant-based protein source and can help maintain healthy blood pressure levels.

- **Greek yogurt:** Greek yogurt is a great source of protein and calcium, which is essential for maintaining healthy bones. It can be a nutritious snack option or an ingredient in recipes.

- **Cauliflower:** Cauliflower is a low-potassium vegetable that can be a substitute for higher potassium vegetables like potatoes. It is also rich in antioxidants and fiber.

- **Cabbage:** Cabbage is a cruciferous vegetable that is low in potassium and high in vitamins K and C. It can be enjoyed raw in salads or cooked in dishes like stir-fries or soups.

- **Berries:** Berries like strawberries, blueberries, and raspberries are not only low in oxalate but also high in antioxidants. They can be enjoyed fresh, frozen, or added to smoothies or oatmeal.

- **Pineapple:** Pineapple contains an enzyme called bromelain, which has anti-inflammatory properties. It can help reduce inflammation in the kidneys and other parts of the body.

- **Seaweed:** Seaweed is a good source of iodine, which is important for maintaining healthy thyroid function. It can be enjoyed in sushi rolls or used as a seasoning in various dishes.

- **Turmeric:** Turmeric contains a compound called curcumin, which has potent anti-inflammatory and antioxidant effects. It can be added to curries, smoothies, or used as a seasoning.

- **Red grapes:** Red grapes contain resveratrol, a compound that has been shown to have protective effects on the kidneys. They can be enjoyed as a snack or used in recipes.

Dark chocolate: Dark chocolate with a high cocoa content contains flavonoids that have antioxidant and anti-inflammatory properties. Moderation is key, but enjoying a small piece of dark chocolate can provide some health benefits.

<u>*Chapter 6*</u>

Meal Planning and Recipes

Creating balanced meals that are kidney stone-friendly involves incorporating a variety of nutrient-rich foods while avoiding those that are high in oxalate, sodium, and animal protein. Here are some tips for meal planning:

1. Start with portion control: Keep an eye on portion sizes to ensure you're not consuming excessive amounts of protein and sodium.

2. Focus on plant-based proteins: Opt for legumes, tofu, tempeh, and Greek yogurt as good sources of protein that are lower in purines and phosphorus.

3. Load up on vegetables: Include a variety of non-oxalate vegetables like cauliflower, cabbage, bell peppers, and carrots. These provide essential nutrients without adding to oxalate levels.

4. Choose whole grains: Instead of refined grains, choose whole grains like quinoa, brown rice, and whole wheat bread for added fiber and nutrients.

5. Incorporate healthy fats: Include foods like avocados, olive oil, and nuts, which are rich in healthy fats like monounsaturated fats and omega-3 fatty acids.

6. Avoid high-oxalate foods: Limit or avoid foods high in oxalate, such as spinach, rhubarb, beets, and almonds. While it's not necessary to completely eliminate these foods, moderation is key.

7. Use herbs and spices: Flavor meals with herbs and spices like turmeric, ginger, basil, and rosemary instead of relying on high-sodium seasonings or sauces.

Sample recipes:

1. Quinoa Salad with Chickpeas and Vegetables:
- Cook 1 cup of quinoa according to package instructions.

- In a large bowl, combine cooked quinoa, 1 can of drained and rinsed chickpeas, sliced cucumbers, cherry tomatoes, diced bell peppers, and chopped parsley.
- In a separate small bowl, whisk together lemon juice, olive oil, minced garlic, and salt to taste. Drizzle over the quinoa mixture and toss to combine. Serve chilled.

2. Grilled Chicken and Vegetable Skewers:
- Cut boneless, skinless chicken breasts into bite-sized pieces.
- In a bowl, marinate the chicken with olive oil, lemon juice, minced garlic, dried oregano, and salt. Let it marinate for at least 30 minutes.
- Preheat the grill to medium heat. Thread the marinated chicken pieces onto skewers alternating with vegetables like bell peppers, red onions, and zucchini.
- Grill the skewers, turning occasionally, until the chicken is cooked through and the vegetables are tender. Serve with a side of quinoa or whole wheat couscous.

3. Greek Yogurt Parfait:
- In a glass or bowl, layer Greek yogurt, fresh berries (such as blueberries or strawberries), and a sprinkle of nuts or granola.
- Repeat the layers until the glass is full.
- Drizzle with a small amount of honey or maple syrup, if desired. Enjoy as a nutritious breakfast or snack.

Certainly! Here are a few more kidney stone-friendly meal ideas:

4. Lentil Soup:
- In a large pot, sauté chopped onions, carrots, and celery in olive oil until tender.
- Add rinsed lentils, vegetable broth, diced tomatoes, and spices like cumin, paprika, and oregano.
- Simmer for about 30-40 minutes until the lentils are cooked through and the flavors are well combined. Serve hot with a side of whole grain bread.

5. Baked Salmon with Roasted Vegetables:
- Preheat the oven to 400°F (200°C). Place salmon fillets on a baking sheet lined with parchment paper or aluminum foil.
- Brush the salmon with a mixture of olive oil, lemon juice, minced garlic, and dill. Season with salt and pepper.
- In a separate bowl, toss mixed vegetables (such as broccoli, cauliflower, and Brussels sprouts) with olive oil, minced garlic, and your choice of herbs. Spread them around the salmon on the baking sheet.
- Bake for about 15-20 minutes until the salmon is cooked through and the vegetables are tender. Serve with a side of quinoa or roasted sweet potatoes.

6. Spinach and Mushroom Omelette:

- In a non-stick skillet, sauté sliced mushrooms and spinach in a small amount of olive oil until wilted. Season with salt and pepper.
- In a separate bowl, whisk together eggs (or egg whites) with a splash of milk or water. Pour the beaten eggs over the sautéed vegetables in the skillet.
- Cook over medium-low heat, lifting the edges of the omelette to allow the uncooked eggs to flow underneath until the eggs are fully set.
- Fold the omelette in half and serve with a side of whole grain toast and fresh fruit.

7. Greek Salad with Grilled Chicken:
- In a bowl, combine chopped romaine lettuce, cucumber slices, cherry tomatoes, diced red onion, Kalamata olives, and crumbled feta cheese.
- Season with salt, pepper, dried oregano, and a drizzle of olive oil and lemon juice.
- Grill chicken breasts until cooked through and slice them into strips. Add the grilled chicken to the salad.
- Serve with a side of whole grain pita bread or quinoa.

8. Quinoa Stuffed Bell Peppers:
- Preheat the oven to 375°F (190°C). Cut the tops off bell peppers and remove the seeds and membranes.
- In a saucepan, cook quinoa according to package instructions.
- In a separate skillet, sauté chopped onions, garlic, and diced mushrooms until they are soft. Add cooked quinoa, diced tomatoes, and your choice of herbs and spices.
- Stuff the bell peppers with the quinoa mixture and place them on a baking dish. Bake for about 25-30 minutes until the peppers are tender.
- Serve with a side salad or steamed vegetables.

9. Shrimp Stir-Fry with Brown Rice:
- In a wok or skillet, heat olive oil and sauté sliced bell peppers, broccoli florets, and snap peas until slightly tender.
- Add peeled and deveined shrimp to the skillet and cook until they turn pink and are cooked through.
- In a small bowl, whisk together low-sodium soy sauce, minced garlic, grated ginger, and a pinch of red pepper flakes. Pour the sauce over the shrimp and vegetables and stir-fry for a few minutes.
- Serve with cooked brown rice.
Remember to make modifications or substitutions based on your own dietary needs and preferences. It's also important to drink plenty of water and stay hydrated to help prevent kidney stone formation.

Chapter 7

PREVALENCE AND IMPACT

Kidney stones are a relatively common condition, with a significant impact on individuals and healthcare systems. Here are some key points regarding their prevalence and impact:

The prevalence of kidney stones is relatively high, with studies suggesting that approximately 1 in 10 people will develop a kidney stone at some point in their lifetime. The incidence of kidney stones has been increasing over the years, likely due to changes in lifestyle, diet, and climate.

Gender and age: Men are more prone to developing kidney stones than women, with a male-to-female ratio of about 3:1. The prevalence tends to peak between the ages of 30 and 60 years but can occur at any age.

Recurrence: Kidney stones have a high recurrence rate. Approximately 50% of individuals who have had a kidney stone will develop another stone within five years if preventive measures are not taken.

Impact on quality of life: Kidney stones can cause severe pain and discomfort, significantly impacting an individual's quality of life. The pain episodes may be debilitating, leading to missed work or reduced productivity. The fear of recurrent stones can also cause anxiety and stress.

Healthcare costs: Kidney stones impose a substantial economic burden on healthcare systems. The costs associated with diagnosis, treatment, and management of kidney stones, including surgical procedures and hospitalizations, can be significant. Additionally, the indirect costs related to lost work hours and decreased productivity further contribute to the overall burden.

Complications and long-term consequences: While most kidney stones pass without causing significant complications, they can lead to various complications such as urinary tract infections, kidney damage, and hydronephrosis. In severe cases, kidney stones may require surgical intervention, which carries its own risks.

Impact on kidney function: Chronic or recurrent kidney stones can, over time, impair kidney function and increase the risk of developing chronic kidney disease (CKD). This highlights the importance of preventive measures and regular monitoring for individuals with a history of kidney stones.

It is crucial to raise awareness about kidney stone prevention strategies, promote early diagnosis, and ensure appropriate management to alleviate the burden of this condition on individuals and healthcare systems.

The impact of kidney stones on individuals can vary depending on the size, location, and number of stones present. Some common symptoms include severe pain in the back or side (referred to as renal colic), blood in the urine, frequent urination, and urinary tract infections.

In addition to the physical discomfort, kidney stones can have several negative consequences on a person's health and quality of life. These can include:

Decreased kidney function: Kidney stones can obstruct the flow of urine, leading to pressure build-up and potential kidney damage. This can reduce kidney function over time if left untreated.

Recurrence: Once a person has had a kidney stone, they are more likely to experience another stone in the future. The risk of recurrence increases if certain underlying medical conditions or dietary factors are present.

Complications: In some cases, kidney stones can cause complications such as hydronephrosis (swelling of the kidney due to urine backup), urinary tract infections, or kidney damage.

Emotional and psychological impact: Dealing with the pain and uncertainty associated with kidney stones can cause stress, anxiety, and depression in some individuals.

Financial burden: Treating kidney stones can be expensive, especially if surgical intervention is required. This can lead to financial strain on individuals and healthcare systems.

Overall, kidney stones can significantly impact a person's well-being, requiring timely diagnosis, appropriate management, and preventive measures to minimize the impact and occurrence of future stones.

Gender differences: Studies have shown that men tend to have a higher incidence of kidney stones compared to women. This could be attributed to hormonal and anatomical differences.

Age distribution: The prevalence of kidney stones tends to peak between the ages of 30 and 50, although they can occur at any age, including in children and older adults.

Impact on daily activities: The pain and discomfort associated with kidney stones can significantly disrupt an individual's daily activities, including work, exercise, and social interactions.

Impact on productivity: Kidney stones can result in missed workdays, reduced work performance, and decreased productivity. This can have economic implications for both individuals and employers.

Health complications: Kidney stones, if not adequately managed, can lead to complications such as chronic kidney disease, kidney damage, or recurrent urinary tract infections.

Dietary factors: Certain dietary habits, such as a diet high in salt, animal protein, and oxalate-rich foods (such as spinach and rhubarb), can increase the risk of developing kidney stones. Modifying dietary intake can play a significant role in prevention and management.

Treatment options: Treatment for kidney stones may include conservative measures (pain medication, increased fluid intake), medications to facilitate stone passage or dissolve stones, or more invasive procedures like extracorporeal shock wave lithotripsy or surgical removal.

Prevention strategies: Adopting lifestyle modifications, such as drinking an adequate amount of water, reducing the intake of certain foods, maintaining a healthy weight, and managing underlying medical conditions, can help prevent the formation of kidney stones.

<u>*Chapter 8*</u>

Fluid Intake Strategies

1. Set a daily goal: Start by setting a goal for how much water you want to consume each day. The general recommendation is to drink at least 8 cups (64 ounces) of fluids, but individual needs may vary.

2. Carry a water bottle: Keep a water bottle with you throughout the day to make it easier to sip on water regularly. Having it nearby will serve as a constant reminder to drink more fluids.

3. Flavor your water: If you find plain water boring, try adding natural flavors such as lemon, lime, cucumber, or mint to enhance the taste. This can make drinking water more enjoyable and encourage higher consumption.

4. Schedule water breaks: Set reminders on your phone or use apps that send you notifications to remind you to drink water throughout the day. Creating a schedule can help you maintain a consistent fluid intake.

5. Keep fluids accessible: Make sure you always have access to fluids by keeping water bottles or other beverages within reach. When fluids are readily available, you are more likely to consume them.

6. Substitute other beverages: Replace sugary or caffeinated drinks like soda, energy drinks, or juices with water. These beverages can increase the risk of kidney stone formation due to their high sugar or oxalate content. Opt for water as a healthier alternative.

7. Eat water-rich foods: Include foods in your diet that have high water content, such as watermelon, cucumbers, oranges, strawberries, and grapefruits. These foods can contribute to your overall fluid intake.

8. Pace yourself: Instead of chugging a large amount of water at once, sip throughout the day. This allows your body to better absorb the fluids and helps prevent feeling overwhelmed by drinking too much water too quickly.

9. Monitor urine color: Use the color of your urine as a guide for hydration. Ideally, your urine should be a light straw color. If it is dark yellow or amber, it may indicate dehydration, and you should drink more fluids.

10. Consult with a healthcare professional: If you are unsure about the ideal fluid intake for your specific needs or have a medical condition, it is best to consult with a healthcare professional. They can provide personalized recommendations based on your health status and help tailor a fluid intake plan for kidney stone prevention.

Certainly! Here are some additional tips to consider for kidney stone prevention through fluid intake:

11. Space out your fluid intake: Rather than consuming most of your fluids at one time, try to spread them out throughout the day. This helps to maintain a steady hydration level and minimize the risk of dehydration.

12. Choose beverages with citric acid: Citric acid can help prevent the formation of certain types of kidney stones. Consider drinking beverages like lemonade or limeade, which naturally contain high levels of citric acid. Alternatively, you can also add a splash of lemon or lime juice to your water.

13. Be mindful of your sodium intake: Higher sodium levels in your diet can contribute to the formation of certain types of kidney stones. Aim to reduce your sodium intake by limiting processed foods, using herbs and spices for flavor instead of salt, and checking food labels for sodium content.

14. Take advantage of herbal teas: Herbal teas such as dandelion tea, nettle tea, or green tea can provide hydration while also offering potential kidney stone prevention benefits. These teas may help with kidney function and have diuretic properties that can increase urine output.

15. Consider the calcium oxalate balance: If you have been advised to limit oxalate intake due to a specific type of kidney stone, it is important to find a balance between calcium and oxalate intake. Low-calcium diets can increase stone risk, so be sure to consult with a healthcare professional or registered dietitian for guidance on appropriate dietary choices.

16. Monitor your fluid intake during exercise or hot weather: It is crucial to increase your fluid intake during periods of intense physical activity or hot weather to compensate for the fluids lost through sweating. Drink water before, during, and after exercise, and consider sports drinks that contain electrolytes if exercising vigorously for more than an hour.

Chapter 9

Frequently Asked Questions

Here are some frequently asked questions and concerns related to diet and kidney stones:

1. Can I still consume calcium if I have kidney stones?

Yes, it's important to consume an adequate amount of calcium, as a low-calcium diet can actually increase the risk of kidney stone formation. However, it's recommended to obtain calcium from food sources rather than supplements. Choose low-fat dairy products or alternatives like fortified plant milk.

2. Are there specific foods I should avoid if I have kidney stones?

The dietary recommendations for kidney stone prevention can vary depending on the type of stone you have. However, there are some general guidelines. It's typically recommended to limit sodium intake, avoid excessive animal protein, and decrease consumption of oxalate-rich foods like spinach, rhubarb, beets, nuts, and chocolate. It's important to work with a healthcare professional or registered dietitian to tailor dietary recommendations to your specific condition and needs.

3. Can I still drink tea or coffee if I have kidney stones?

Tea and coffee, especially certain types like black tea and instant coffee, can contain high amounts of oxalates. If you have a history of calcium oxalate stones, it may be beneficial to limit your consumption of these beverages or opt for lower oxalate alternatives.

4. How much fluid should I drink to prevent kidney stones?

Staying hydrated is crucial for kidney stone prevention. Aim to drink at least 8 cups (64 ounces) of water per day. However, fluid needs can vary depending on factors such as activity level, climate, and individual health conditions. It's a good idea to consult with a healthcare professional or registered dietitian to determine the appropriate fluid intake for your specific needs.

5. Can I still enjoy certain types of fruits and vegetables if I have kidney stones?

Yes, most fruits and vegetables are generally healthy to consume, even if you're at risk for kidney stones. However, if you have a specific type of stone, such as a calcium oxalate stone, it may be necessary to limit intake of high-oxalate fruits and vegetables. Again, it's important to work with a healthcare professional or registered dietitian to determine which foods are best suited for your condition.

6. Can I drink alcohol if I have kidney stones?

Excessive alcohol consumption can dehydrate the body, which can increase the risk of kidney stones. It's generally recommended to moderate or avoid alcohol to maintain proper hydration and minimize the risk of stone formation.

7. Can I eat dairy products if I have kidney stones?

Yes, you can consume dairy products if you have kidney stones. In fact, including adequate amounts of calcium-rich foods in your diet, such as low-fat dairy products, can help prevent certain types of kidney stones. However, it's important to discuss your specific dietary needs and restrictions with a healthcare professional or registered dietitian, as recommendations may vary depending on the type of stone you have.

8. Does drinking lemonade help prevent kidney stones?

Drinking lemonade, specifically lemon juice, may help prevent kidney stones in some cases. Lemon juice contains citrate, a compound that can help inhibit the formation of calcium-based stones. It's believed that citrate can help prevent the aggregation of crystals that form stones. However, it's important to work with a healthcare professional or registered dietitian to determine the appropriate amount of lemonade or lemon juice to consume for kidney stone prevention.

9. Are there any specific supplements or vitamins that can help prevent kidney stones?

There are certain supplements or vitamins that may be recommended for kidney stone prevention depending on your specific situation. For example, if you have a history of calcium oxalate stones, your healthcare professional or registered dietitian may recommend vitamin B6 supplementation, as it can help decrease oxalate production. However, it's important to note that these recommendations will vary based on individual needs, and you should always consult with a healthcare professional before starting any supplements or vitamins.

10. Can weight loss or dieting affect the risk of developing kidney stones?

Weight loss or strict dieting can potentially increase the risk of developing kidney stones. Rapid weight loss can lead to dehydration, and this lack of proper hydration can increase the likelihood of stone formation. If you're trying to lose weight, it's important to do so in a healthy and gradual manner while maintaining proper hydration.

It's crucial to consult with a healthcare professional or registered dietitian for personalized advice on diet and lifestyle changes to prevent kidney stones. They can evaluate your specific situation, medical history, and stone composition to provide appropriate recommendations.

11. Are all kidney stones the same?

No, kidney stones can vary in terms of their composition. The most common types of kidney stones include calcium oxalate stones, which are formed when calcium and oxalate combine in the urine, and uric acid stones, which are formed from the excessive excretion of uric acid. There are also other less common types of kidney stones, such as struvite stones (related to urinary tract infections) and cystine stones (related to an inherited disorder). The type of stone a person has can determine the recommended treatment and preventive measures.

12. Can certain beverages increase the risk of kidney stones?

Yes, certain beverages may increase the risk of kidney stones. Beverages that are high in oxalate, such as tea, chocolate milk, and dark-colored sodas, can contribute to the formation of calcium oxalate stones. Additionally, excessive consumption of sugary drinks and sodas can lead to weight gain and dehydration, which can increase the risk of stone formation. It is generally recommended to limit or moderate the intake of these beverages, especially for individuals with a history of kidney stones.

13. Is it possible for kidney stones to pass on their own?

Yes, small kidney stones can often pass on their own without medical intervention. If the stone is small enough (usually less than 5mm), the person may experience pain as the stone moves through the urinary tract and eventually passes out of the body. Drinking plenty of water and staying adequately hydrated can help facilitate this process. However, if the stone is larger or causing severe symptoms, medical intervention may be necessary to remove or break up the stone.

14. Can stress contribute to the formation of kidney stones?

While stress itself may not directly cause kidney stones, it can contribute to certain lifestyle factors that increase the risk. For example, when people are stressed, they may be more likely to consume unhealthy foods, engage in poor dietary habits, or neglect proper hydration. These factors can all contribute to the formation of kidney stones. Managing stress through healthy coping mechanisms, such as exercise, relaxation techniques, and seeking support, can help reduce the risk of stone formation.

15. Are there any specific foods that should be avoided to prevent kidney stones?

Certain foods may be recommended to avoid or limit in order to prevent kidney stones, depending on the type of stone a person is prone to. For example, individuals with calcium oxalate stones may be advised to limit their intake of high-oxalate foods like spinach, rhubarb, and beets. Those with uric acid stones may be advised to reduce their consumption of purine-rich foods like organ meats and shellfish. However, recommendations can vary based on individual needs, and it's important to consult with a healthcare professional or registered dietitian for personalized dietary advice.

Remember, these answers are general and may not apply to everyone. Always consult with a healthcare professional or registered dietitian for personalized advice based on your specific medical condition.

Chapter 10

Conclusion

In concluding "Everything to Know About Kidney Stones," this comprehensive guide has embarked on a thorough expedition into the realm of kidney stones. By dissecting their origins, risk factors, and treatment avenues, the book has illuminated a path toward understanding and managing this common medical challenge. With its amalgamation of medical insights and practical advice, readers are now equipped with the tools to navigate their own journeys, armed with awareness and strategies to prevent and alleviate the discomfort caused by kidney stones. This book stands as an indispensable resource, fostering a future of informed decisions and improved kidney health.

Disclaimer:
The information provided in this book, "Everything to Know About Kidney Stones," is intended for educational and informational purposes only. While every effort has been made to ensure the accuracy and reliability of the content, the author and publisher are not responsible for any errors or omissions, or for any consequences arising from the use of the information provided herein. Readers are advised to consult with qualified medical professionals for personalized guidance and treatment options related to kidney stones or any other health concerns. The author and publisher disclaim any liability for the decisions and actions taken by readers based on the information presented in this book.

www.ingramcontent.com/pod-product-compliance
Lightning Source LLC
Chambersburg PA
CBHW080855250726
48663CB00004B/474